Dedicated
to
finding the courage
and strength
to
"CHANGE"

Paperback ISBN: 979-8-9927261-0-7
E-book ISBN: 979-8-9927261-1-4

Copyright© Jeff Shammah 2025
All rights reserved, including the right
of reproduction in whole or in part in any form.

Choosing: A Healthy Lifestyle

(Taking Action!)

By Jeff Shammah

Simplicity

Books on Exercise are:

1. Short and easy to read.

2. Change-the need and necessity of it throughout life.

3. Less is more / **Quality** over Quantity.

4. Copying-be inspired by, but do not copy the routines of others (one size does not fit all).

5. Think-for yourself, be **MINDFUL**, find a teacher (guidance), and put in the **WORK** in order to find your own exercise prescription.

6. Reference Tool-to be read and re-read throughout your life in order to **GROW WITH YOU**.

7. Long term results instead of **TEMPORARY RESULTS**.

Universal Principle

We "Human Beings" are too complex to be placed in a category.

Our diversity and our complexity require Individual Health Prescriptions.

The Beginning

Through the books:

Exercise. Why? (Book 1), ***How?*** (Book 2), and ***What?*** (Book 3),

you learned of the importance of **EXERCISE** and the need to AVOID ONE-SIZE-FITS-ALL programs for **YOUTH, MIDDLE AGE,** and **ADVANCED AGE.** Instead, working towards an **INDIVIDUAL HEALTH PRESCRIPTION.** Which will help you to develop tools and coping skills needed; in order to protect yourself mentally, physically and emotionally throughout life's inevitable ups and downs.

In my career as a personal trainer, I've worked with and seen, human beings challenged by life **REGARDLESS OF AGE:**

Youth-
puberty, social media, and the sense of invincibility and immortality.

Middle Age-
at a crossroads, dealing with confusion and midlife crisis.

Advanced Age-
aging, feeling invisible, and the loss of self worth.

Life, is not necessarily fair. So those who are challenged the most: Genetic Defects, Life Threatening Illness, Poverty, and Prejudice. Will need to work even harder to maintain a **HEALTHY BALANCED LIFESTYLE.** Whether we, **HUMANITY,** are out of balance (unfit), or the **EARTH** through climate change (unhealthy), we still have a choice-

Give up or fight back?

By making healthier choices and choosing a healthier lifestyle, it will improve our **STRENGTH, ENDURANCE,** and **MENTAL CLARITY,** in dealing with life's many challenges. We have **EVOLVED** from hunter gatherers (active lifestyles) to technologically advanced (sedentary lifestyles). We can either become **BENEFICIARIES** of technology, and use it wisely to help solve life's problems and improve efficiency. Or, we can become **VICTIMS** of technology by not taking the time to:

Stop, slowdown, breathe, stretch, eat and drink nutritionally, love and sleep.

Choosing a healthy lifestyle is **MUCH MORE** than an exercise, a food, or a trend. It is the decision to come face to face with **ONESELF.** Our strengths, our weaknesses, our fears, and our vulnerabilities. It is accepting responsibility for **YOUR OWN HEALTH.** Otherwise, depending on the state of your health, we become vulnerable to:

- marketing ploys
- extreme nutritional advice
- unhealthy trends
- exaggerated promises of results

Once we choose to better understand ourselves and incorporate our self awareness (truth), we can then begin the process of **FORGIVING OURSELVES** (based on perceived weaknesses), and improving our health.

Not looking for convenience and instant gratification, but **LONG-TERM LIFESTYLE CHANGES** and **RESULTS.**

Now, we take action!

Taking Action!

In order to "thrive"
(flourish or grow vigorously)
as human beings, we need and require a healthy exposure to:

Love - of self, family, and others.

Sleep - establishing regular sleep cycles.

Nutrition - fuel.

Work - purpose and responsibility.

Exercise - movement and self maintenance.

Music - our spiritual connection to the universe.

Dance - our self expression of our spirit.

Art - our physical creation of the spirit.

Nature - fresh air, life giving growth, and our most basic and primal self.

Meditation - self discovery and self understanding.

"In order to be truly healthy"

Love

Taking care of your mental, emotional, and physical **"SELF"** through exercise, is a sign of self love and an appreciation for the GIFT OF LIFE. It says to your **FAMILY,** I will be capable of being there for you when needed.

It is the demonstration of the respect for **OTHERS** around you, and the wish to be your **BEST SELF** while sharing life with them.

> An appreciation *for the* gift of life.

Sleep

Sleep allows you to recuperate from the stress of raising a family, work, exercise, and socializing with others; and **RECUPERATION** is the key to results.

While sleeping, our **BRAIN** and **BODY** are cleansed, muscle, bone, and tissue repaired. Mental and emotional issues are worked out, all in preparation for the next day. Establishing **REGULAR SLEEP CYCLES** and **HEALTHY SLEEPING PATTERNS** over a 24 hour cycle (circadian rhythm), and allowing for proper **HORMONAL BALANCE,** is crucial to good health.

Obviously being a new parent and taking care of a baby, as well as life's emergencies, will make this difficult and at times impossible. But being aware of the importance of sleep, and planning and improving upon the number of hours, meal times, mattress, pillow and environmental conditions (limiting exposure to technological devices/dark window shades); before going to bed will help.

As well as speaking with your doctor or sleep specialist, when necessary.

Nutrition

All health professionals (especially nutritionists) learn about the body's need for nutrition (fuel).

Macronutrients- carbohydrates (simple/complex), fats (saturated/unsaturated), and protein (animal/plant).

Micronutrients- vitamins, minerals, water etc.

Each have a unique function, and play a vital role in your body's health. The body cannot function properly without **ALL OF THEM**. Choosing one over the other is misleading and potentially dangerous.

Examples of exceptions are:

- Allergic reactions to foods
- Diabetes, digestive disorders, intolerances
- Religious, traditional and personal beliefs
- Climate fears

Nutrition will affect your:

- **Metabolism-** raise it or lower it, depending upon proper meal intervals (times) and volume of food.

- **Blood Sugar-** raise it or lower it, depending on **WHAT** you eat, and intervals (times).

- **Mood and Behavior-** processed, high sugar, high fat, and high sodium foods, can lead to mood swings and a change in our behavior.

- **Quality of Sleep-** too much alcohol, soda, caffeine, and overeating just before bedtime, can interrupt sleep.

- **Exercise Results-** without proper nutrition, the body cannot repair and rebuild muscle tissue. Rehydrate, and regulate PH and fluid balance (acidity/alkalinity).

- **Improper weight gain/weight loss-** either too much or too fast. Leading to dangerous health issues and **LACK OF LONG TERM RESULTS.**

- Water- after oxygen, it is the second most important nutrient. It affects and is involved in every process that the body goes through. Maintaining proper hydration is key to a healthy mind and body.

Start your day with a glass of water, nutritious breakfast, then coffee (not on an empty stomach).

When making the decision on how to properly **FUEL** your body and respect your individual needs, talking to a certified **NUTRITIONIST** will help.

> Water *is the second most* important nutrient.

Work

Work helps instill discipline, and provides us with **PURPOSE** and **RESPONSIBILITY**.

When applied to every aspect of our lives:

- HEALTH
- FAMILY
- EMPLOYMENT
- CARING FOR OTHERS
- ENVIRONMENT

It allows us to reach our full potential.

There are a lot of individuals with potential...but few who realize their full potential.

The difference between saying I can do something, and actually doing it...

is realized action!

Exercise

Having worked with individuals throughout decades of their lives, on a weekly basis, **REALITY SETS IN.** That being able to maintain one's health requires a **VARIETY** of ways and **TECHNIQUES,** that **CHANGE** according to the **SITUATION, AGE, ILLNESS,** and **INJURY,** of the individual. We should never exercise outside, in a gym, or at home, without **FIRST** being **MINDFUL** of this. Exercising without previous thought or plan, and choosing any piece of equipment at the gym; is like choosing any doctor at a hospital, instead of the one specific to your needs.

The way that our General Practitioner (primary care doctor) guides us and recommends a **SPECIALIST** when needed; a Personal Trainer guides you on the proper choice of exercise and use of equipment.

This proper choice of exercise, now more than ever, needs modification. Because of the **OVERUSE OF TECHNOLOGY.** The seated, hunched over posture, and repetitive use of the shoulders, hands and fingers. Often leads to **EYE, NECK, SHOULDER, ARM, WRIST** and **FINGER** problems.

Emphasizing the need for "Postural Exercises":

• **A Strong Core** - abdominal, lower back, and gluteal muscles.

• **Movement and Stretching** - to restore neck, shoulder, back, hip, and groin flexibility. And, counteract the sedentary lifestyle and frozen joints that come from a limited range of motion.

• **Glute (buttocks),
Pulling and Backward Strengthening Exercises**

- Glute bridges, squats, lunges, pliés, and leg lifts.
- Lowerback: airplane, swimmer, and superman lifts.
- Upperback: lat pulldowns, pull ups, chin ups and dumbell rows.
- Shoulder: Rear Deltoid backward lateral raises.

• Abdominal Muscles

- **Rectus abdominus** (center) holds internal organs in place and stabilizes body during movement.

- **Pyramidalis** (base of pubic bone) helps maintain internal pressure.

- **External obliques** (sides towards middle) allows trunk of body to twist from side to side.

- **Internal obliques** (lateral side of abdomen just inside hip bone) aids in twisting and turning.

- **Transversus abdominis** (deepest, below internal and external obliques) helps in stabilizing trunk and maintaining internal abdominal pressure.

These strong bands of muscles lining the walls of your abdomen, help protect your **SPINE**. Maintain **POSTURE, BALANCE,** and resist the **NEGATIVE EFFECTS** of **GRAVITY** pushing down on us overtime.

> Proper guidance is NECESSARY,
> on CHOICE and USE,
> of abdominal exercises.
> In order to
> AVOID STRAINS and HERNIAS.

- **Strength Training**-weight lifting:
  - to reduce **MUSCLE LOSS** (atrophy/sarcopenia)
  - slowdown **BONE DENSITY LOSS** (osteoperosis)
  - raise **METABOLISM**
  - improve **BODY COMPOSITION** (ratio of muscle to fat)

- **Cardio**
  - strengthening the **HEART MUSCLE** (organ)
  - **CARDIOVASCULAR SYSTEM** (blood vessels and their elasticity)
  - improving **MAXIMAL OXYGEN UPTAKE** (V02 max)

There are many options:

Calisthenics (bodyweight)
Yoga, martial arts, gymnastics, dance, boxing, ballet, swimming, running, cycling, rowing, hiking, climbing, walking, etc.

Free Weights (functional equipment)
Barbells, dumbells, kettlebells, rubber bands, stability balls, balance boards, etc.

Machines
For safety and ease of use (leg press, lat pulldown, etc.)

Your choice of exercise program needs to contain the 7 Components of Physical Fitness:

1. Muscular Strength
The amount of weight you can lift or move with maximum force, for a **SHORT** period of time.

2. Muscular Endurance
Repeated contractions against a load (weight) for an **EXTENDED** period of time.

3. Flexibility
Range of motion of your joints.

4. Balance
Equal distribution of weight.

5. Coordination
The ability to use different parts of the body together, smoothly, and efficiently.

6. Agility (nimbleness)
An ability to change the body's position quickly and easily.

7. Speed
The act or state of moving swiftly (velocity), or rate of performance.

And the variables affecting these components and type of exercise:

Intensity (how hard)
Your heart rate, perceived exertion, or resistance level.

Duration (how long)
Total time spent exercising, in a single session.

Frequency (how often)
The number of times you exercise per week.

Recovery (modalities)
Sleep, massage, hot and cold therapies, ointments, foam roller and balls, meditation, etc.

> All applied in a
> **PROGRESSIVE, CONSISTENT** and
> **PATIENT** manner.

Guidance and instruction on their use, from an **ACCREDITED** (licensed/certified) and **EXPERIENCED** teacher is **NECESSARY**. In learning how to **PROPERLY** and **SAFELY** exercise.

Music

Whether listening to, dancing to, singing to, playing, composing or conducting. **MUSIC IS OUR SPIRITUAL CONNECTION TO THE UNIVERSE.** Its vibrational force and sound, has the power to lift or lower our spirits, unite or separate us, instill fear or evoke (bring or recall) great joy. Understood and used throughout the world for **COMMUNICATING, HEALING,** and **ENHANCING HEALTH.**

> Music is our spiritual connection to the universe

Dance

OUR SELF EXPRESSION OF SPIRIT.

Used to pay homage and respect to our ancestors.

To communicate stories and give messages.

For self defense and sharing. A form of

MENTAL, EMOTIONAL, and **PHYSICAL** release.

A practice throughout the world that touches an innate

(inborn/natural) need and response from us.

Dance is our self expression of spirit

Art

Observing it, creating it, being inspired or emotionally moved by it. It has the power to communicate and tell stories.

ART IS OUR PHYSICAL CREATION OF THE SPIRIT.

Art is our physical creation of the spirit.

Nature

Mountains, Oceans, Rivers,

Trees, Plants, Animals, Insects, etc.

- Fresh Air
- Life Giving Growth

and...

- Our Most Basic,

"Primal Self"

Nature is
our most basic
"Primal Self"

Meditation

Making the time for:

- Quietude (calmness)
- Internal "self" conversation
- Stillness

will lead towards **"SELF DISCOVERY"** and **"SELF UNDERSTANDING"**.

Meditation is
our path towards
self discovery
and understanding.

Breathing, Meditation and Exercise

For far too long, individuals have chosen either **MIND** (cerebral) or **BODY** (physical).

IT NEEDS TO BE BOTH (nervous system) in order for us to be balanced, healthy human beings.

The practice of breathing in various postures through **MOTION** and **MOTIONLESS** exercises; allows our **BRAIN** and **BODY** to reboot, recharge, strengthen, and cleanse.

Therefore, function better.

This includes:

- General breathing at rest.
- Giving birth, athletic breaths, singing (an enormous unleashing of power).
- Respiratory diseases and illness (asthma/COPD)
- Meditative breaths (hard and soft).

There is **NO "ONE RIGHT WAY"** to breathe. It depends on the circumstance, system, technique, and the person. What matters most is that we find a qualified experienced teacher to show us how, and guide us towards improving our breathing.

Human Tree

Nurturing, Nourishing, Exercise, Meditation

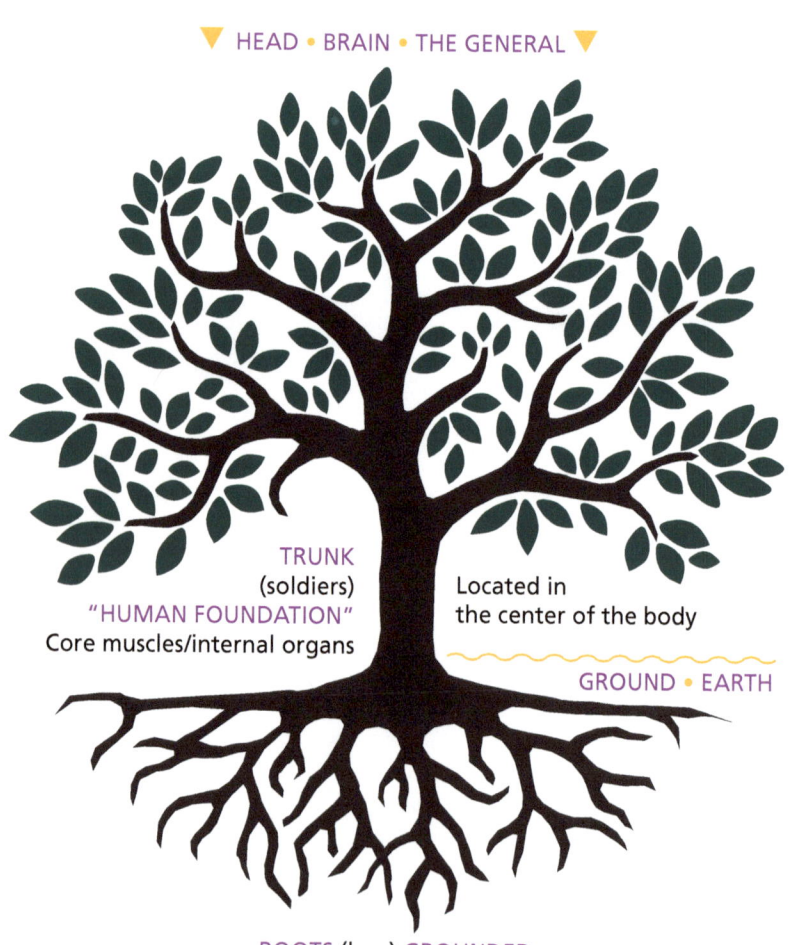

The **TREE** (human) is one of life's greatest examples for us to learn from and emulate, when performing our exercises.

To be **SIMULTANEOUSLY** grounded (legs) to the earth, while growing upward through the **TRUNK** (core), and expanding outward (head and arms) to the sky.

So begin "taking action" to **INCORPORATE** a little bit of each of these into your life, and enjoy the JOURNEY TO BETTER HEALTH!

Enjoy the journey to better health!

Observations

concerning

Exercise

and

Health

Secrets

There are NO "secret foods" or "secret exercises". What works for one person, does not necessarily work for another. What worked for one period of time in life, will not necessarily work for another period of time in life.

Looking for these is lazy and potentially dangerous to your health. Instead, choose a well rounded and balanced approach for your health routine.

Including a **LARGE VARIETY OF WHOLE FOODS** (minimally processed foods, close to their natural form). Always taking into account your individual needs, allergies, and tolerances.

Remain **OPEN MINDED** to **ALL FORMS OF EXERCISE** and their proper use.

Continuing to learn about what to **ADD** and what to **REMOVE**, from your routine **AS YOU AGE**.

Golden Age

Wisdom is the proper use of experience (Book 1).

"We really are what we think". Focus on what you have gained (positive). NOT, on what you have lost (negative).

In order to:

- Stand and walk (back pain, sciatica).
- Play with your grandchildren, and participate in their lives.
- Maintain your **INDEPENDENCE**, and open up **NEW CHAPTERS** (hobbies) in your life.

Takes great energy!

As opposed to a depressing, sedentary, lonely lifestyle. This will require the **RE-AWAKENING** of the **CHILD WITHIN**. But, with wisdom, experience, and knowledge.

Make sure that you find a teacher experienced enough to work with older individuals. **ABLE TO MODIFY** the exercises, and **GRADUALLY** build up your ability to perform fully.

Not one size fits all.

Body Alignment
and Weight Distribution

- When carrying bags, try to distribute the weight evenly on both sides of the body. Instead of carrying everything on one side of your body. IF NOT, this will, over time (years), lead to misalignment and poor posture as we age.

- Favorite chair or couch (at home)-center yourself while watching television, using technology, or reading. Focus on proper alignment, posture, and support of your spine.

In order to avoid the formation, over time, of bad postural habits and joint pain.

- Address Foot issues-wear proper shoes, sneakers, and slippers, according to your individual needs. Whether your feet are prone to:

  - *Inversion* (foot turns inward).
  - *Eversion* (foot turns outward).
  - *Supination* (foot rolls outward).
  - *Pronation* (foot rolls inward).
  - *Flat Feet* (tendon issues/ligament issues/fallen arches).

In order to avoid future problems with your feet, ankles, knees, and back.

Speaking to and working with a **PODIATRIST** (foot doctor), in order to assess your foot mechanics and recommend appropriate treatment options, is necessary.

For total body alignment and re-alignment (musculoskeletal) conditions and treatments, speaking to and working with a licensed **CHIROPRACTOR** or **ALIGNMENT SPECIALIST,** for answers and guidance, is necessary.

Quick

Weight Loss or Gain (using shortcuts).

Using **DRUGS** or **EXTREME DIETS** without proper guidance and supervision from your doctor or a nutritionist, can increase the potential for DANGEROUS SIDE EFFECTS TO YOUR HEALTH AND INTERNAL ORGANS.

And, it still does not address the 7 components of physical fitness. Muscular strength, muscular endurance, flexibility, balance, coordination, agility and speed.

Often leading to even **MORE WEIGHT GAIN** later, or illness.

> Proper guidance and supervision *from a professional* is necessary.

Dental Hygiene

Proper care and maintenance of your **TEETH** and **MOUTH** are crucial to your total wellbeing.

> *Guidance and care from your* Dentist *is necessary.*

Form and Progressions

At any stage of your health routine: starting/beginner, recuperating from illness, or injury.

You do not go 100%!

Instead, you should improve through stages (progressions).

In order to obtain **LONG LASTING RESULTS** and AVOID INJURY, it is necessary to use **PROPER FORM** and **PROGRESSIONS**.

Practiced over several months and years. NOT, DAYS AND WEEKS.

Genetics

Often, individuals purchase or copy another persons exercise routine. Thinking that they will look like them. Copying your favorite persons workout, **WILL NOT** give you their body (genetics). You can only improve within your individual potential.

But, everyone can improve their health, looks, and how they feel.

GENETICS and **INDIVIDUALITY** will take precedence.

Instead, use them for **INSPIRATION** and **GUIDANCE,** on how to reach **YOUR INDIVIDUAL POTENTIAL.**

Recuperation

(Book 1)

Yes, you can overdo anything!

As we advance through life, **"MORE OF EVERYTHING"** does not necessarily translate into greater results. But often:

Burn out, Imbalance and Unhappiness.

Learn to work **SMARTER** and **MORE EFFICIENTLY** through proper **RECUPERATION** (nutrition and sleep). In order to achieve **"CLARITY"** and make wiser choices.

We, as Human Beings, do not need to like exercise. But, we need to understand the necessity of exercise.

There is very little, or nothing, a person can do:

- We cannot take care of our **SELF** or **FAMILY**.
- We cannot go to **WORK**.
- We cannot **SOCIALIZE**.

...if we are **OFTEN SICK** or **HOSPITALIZED**.

> Exercise *is required* in order to *move* and *function well.*

Obstacles

*(to our growth)
and*

"Convenient Amnesia"

It is said that:

We hear what we want to hear...
We see what we want to see...

"Convenient Amnesia"

(choosing to ignore what is right in front of us,
and purposefully forget past lessons).

How do we break this cycle?

We will need to master the ability to **SLOW THINGS DOWN** (meditation). A skill that needs to be practiced.

STILLNESS-when we are incapable of being still:
- Listening and paying attention
- Observing and admiring landscapes (nature)
- Sleeping and recuperating
- **MEDITATION**

It is a sign of **IMBALANCE** in the **NERVOUS SYSTEM** (mind and body).

The **"HUMAN BODY"** when properly functioning,
does not need EXCESSIVE use of:

- Technology
- **Caffeine, Energy Drinks, Drugs, Alcohol** or **Junk Food**

The **OVERUSE** of these, is a sign of imbalanced living. Too much of one thing (stress), and not enough of the other (recovery).

EXTREME BEHAVIOR creates **EXTREME RESPONSES** by the body. And, extreme behavior comes from a lack of **BALANCE**, and a lack of **PREVENTION**.

TAKING ACTION does not mean waiting for someone else to give us all of the answers. It is accepting responsibility for our own health, and properly using all of the **HEALTH PROFESSIONALS** to help guide us along the way.

Not pointing the finger...**but instead looking within.**

When an individual is finally ready to change:

They will hear what was actually said...
Not what they chose to hear.

They will see what is actually there...
Not what they chose to see.

And above all, listen first and foremost to their "Inner Voice", that knows the **TRUTH**. Rather than justify or make excuses.

As the **FADS** and **TRENDS COME** and **GO** in exercise. We will not fall backwards, but instead, make sense of all the **OPTIONS** and **CHOICES** in exercise programs available.

Thereby allowing ourselves to make better choices, and to experience LASTING RESULTS and **LONGEVITY**. With a more BALANCED and HOLISTIC approach to HEALTH.

> Above all, *listen to the "Inner Voice" that knows* the truth.

Acknowledgment

To know something...
is to do it *(practice)* in your daily life.

Not talking about it, talk is cheap *(easy),* doing is challenging *(work).*

In order to be **SELF EMPOWERED,** to give **ONESELF** credit for growth and improvement,

"You need to do the work".

Self confidence (self esteem) is manufactured through the effort we make to search for, practice, and learn as we grow. NOT, by looking for someone to give us all of the answers. But instead, to be inspired by others, learn from others, NOT copy others.

It is the individual CHOOSING TO TAKE ACTION, and live a more healthy, satisfying, and love filled existence.

And then, choosing to SHARE that ENRICHMENT with OTHERS.

To be continued...

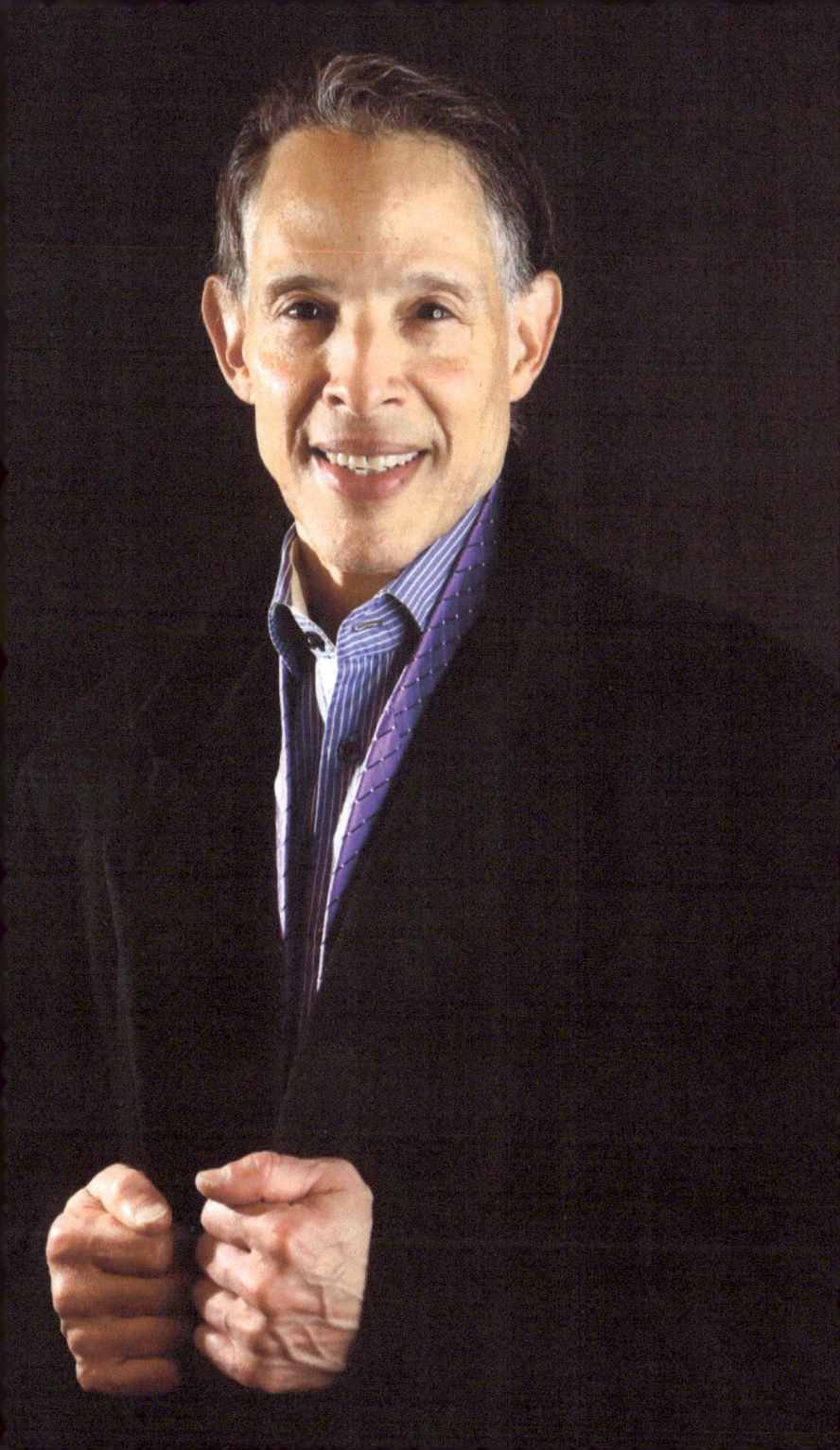

Credits

Photography
Susie Lang

Design
Jeffrey Shammah with Gloria Gregurovich

www.ingramcontent.com/pod-product-compliance
Lightning Source LLC
Chambersburg PA
CBHW040934030426
42337CB00001B/9

9798992726107